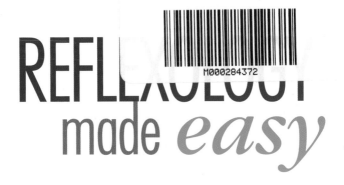

REFLEXOLOGY
made *easy*

Self-help Techniques for **Everyday** Ailments

Ewald Kliegel

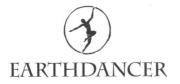

EARTHDANCER

A FINDHORN PRESS IMPRINT

Disclaimer

The information in this book is given in good faith and is neither intended to diagnose any physical or mental condition nor to serve as a substitute for informed medical advice or care.

Please contact your health professional for medical advice and treatment. Neither author nor publisher can be held liable by any person for any loss or damage whatsoever which may arise from the use of this book or any of the information therein.

First edition 2015

Reflexology made easy
Ewald Kliegel

Cover photography: Fred Hageneder
Models: Eliza Misu, Jens Jacobsen
Illustrations: © Ewald Kliegel

This English edition © 2015 Earthdancer GmbH
English translation © JMS books llp
Editing by JMS books llp (www.jmseditorial.com)
Original title published in German as *Reflexzonen Easy*
World copyright © 2014 Neue Erde GmbH
All rights reserved

Cover design: Dragon Design
Set in News Gothic
Typesetting and graphic design: Dragon Design

Printed and bound in China by Midas Printing Ltd.

ISBN 978-1-84409-666-4

Published by Earthdancer GmbH, an imprint of:
Findhorn Press, 117-121 High Street,
Forres, IV36 1AB, Scotland.
www.earthdancerbooks.com,
www.findhornpress.com

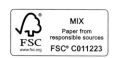

MIX
Paper from
responsible sources
FSC® C011223

Contents

Important notice and treatment restrictions

Reflex zone massage (reflexology) can be enjoyed at any age, although you should ensure that the treatments are always enjoyable and never become painful. If a reflex zone produces a sensitive reaction, it is best to adapt and reduce the intensity of the technique.

Certain restrictions have to be applied to every effective technique, and reflexology is no exception. Massages should be administered during pregnancy only with the unequivocal consent of a doctor, and even then all abdominal and hormone-related zones must be avoided. Reflex zone massage must not be used in cases of serious illness, such as cancer, chronic rheumatism, illness where fever is present or conditions that are acutely debilitating. And all symptoms of illness that cannot be explained must be referred to a medical professional. Please also be aware that reflexology treatment can enhance the effects of medicines.

Foreword

Be honest. What sort of ailments and problems make you visit the doctor? Is a slight headache enough, or do you wait until it's a chronic migraine? And what about that feeling of tightness or stiffness in the joints when the weather changes, or a cold or muscle tension? As a rule, we manage without a doctor for these kinds of annoying but common small complaints. Some people just say to themselves 'it'll be fine', while others pop a few tablets; but there's a third option, one that allows us to exploit the communication channels between the surface of the skin and the inner organs: reflexology. Applying pressure briefly to the head will make the feet feel warm; a few massage strokes on the hands will relieve lower abdominal tension during menstruation; and self-massage of the lower back will improve circulation in the legs when travelling by plane.

So is reflexology some kind of new miracle therapy? Not at all! It is, however, a convincingly effective technique with a long history and has proved its considerable worth in both everyday and therapeutic contexts. Whether you are at home, in the car or at a party, your reflex zones are tools for preventative health care and can boost your powers of self-healing in all kinds of situations in life. An added bonus with these applications is that they can be combined with many other techniques and physiotherapy treatment is significantly more effective when used in conjunction with reflex zone massage, for example, and essential oils, coloured light and crystals lend the technique an extra dimension, greatly extending the effectiveness of a wide range of treatments.

During times when the healthcare sector is forced to make economies, every step towards taking personal responsibility for our health is a step in the right direction. Making use of the reflex zones is without doubt one of the steps we should be taking as it trains us to pay more attention to ourselves, and in this capacity, the zones can be used as preventative measures, helping us to sidestep difficulties and lessening the severity of bouts of illness.

Most importantly, we always have the tools we need to hand, quite literally: our hands (for massage) and the surface of our skin, where all our many reflex zones are to be found. A knowledge of the zones should therefore be a part of every 'first aid manual'.

Wishing you joy and the very best of luck with your reflex zones,

Ewald Kliegel

Our health maps

Most people have heard of the reflex zones, but treating them is often viewed as an old and over-complicated Chinese technique. No surprise then that reflexology has yet to become mainstream.

However, the principle of the reflex zones is quite simple and the system is easy to follow. Imagine that, when complications arise, your body's organs can switch on a warning light, like on the dashboard of a car, as a kind of visual diagnostic tool showing what is wrong. Reflex zones are the error indicators that pop up on our own 'dashboard' that is with us at all times: our skin. These 'emergency signals' appear on the skin in the form of reddening, swelling, spots or eczema, to name just a few of these signs.

Tuck into the meat dishes at a boozy dinner, and the liver and gall bladder are pushed to their limits and the emergency signals or 'warning lights' appear in the form of swelling around the liver and gall bladder zones of the various reflex zone systems, such as on the feet or back. The next day, blemishes may even appear in the relevant zones on the skin of the face. In this way, the reflex zones are an external indication that something is not right internally. When these kinds of symptoms appear, it is no wonder that attempts to treat them cosmetically achieve little; however, when support is provided for the organs affected, the skin problems clear up on their own – when the oil indicator light goes on on the dashboard of a car, we check the oil, we don't disconnect the indicator light. In the case of overindulgence in meat dishes, suitable complementary treatments would include – in addition to reflex zone massage – drinking herbal teas with bitter compounds and avoiding fat and alcohol to relieve the pressure on the liver. This allows the organs to then switch off their warning lights.

Reflex zone signs at a glance

The signs or symptoms on the left suggest the conclusions drawn about the condition of the connective tissue in the associated organs listed on the right:

Reddening and sensitive zones	The organ has excess energy
Swelling	Usually, irritation arising from hyperacidity in the connective tissue
Spots	A build-up of waste products in the organ's connective tissue; spots are a way of indicating this pressure
Eczema	The connective tissue has been massively overstimulated – seek professional advice.
Pale zones	The organ has insufficient energy
Retraction	This area is significantly undersupplied with energy
Nodules	Metabolic waste products are being deposited in the connective tissue
Warts	Emotional strain – take note of what the organ is trying to tell you

These emergency signals or 'warning lights' alone would justify the reflex zones' reputation as a 'health map', but they are capable of even more. In addition to identifying problems, most of the zones also allow us to exert an influence on our body's functions. This opens up an absolute gold mine of applications, with a wide range of options for therapists and professionals offering wellbeing treatments, as well as lay practitioners.

Reflex zones have proved their effectiveness; the German physiotherapist Elisabeth Dicke was able to save her leg from amputation in 1928 by intensively massaging those on her back on a daily basis. Her connective tissue massage technique has since been adopted in the syllabus for masseurs and physiotherapists. At the same time, the physician Ferdinand Huneke was also making use of the reflex zones on the back in his neural therapy, which has found favour with doctors and alternative practitioners ever since.

The best-known zones (on the feet) also have an impressive track record of success: once decoded by American physician Dr William Fitzgerald at the end of the 19th century, they soon began their triumphal march around the world. Treatment of the foot reflex zones was the most common therapy in New York as early as 1900, and, one hundred years later, the first scientific attempts are now being made to investigate the millions of successful treatments achieved using the reflex zones. University lecturer Dr Erich Mur and his team at the University of Innsbruck were able to prove in a 1999 study that blood circulation in the kidneys rose significantly after massage of the kidney zones on the feet, while massage of the head zones in the control group revealed no effect on the kidneys. In 2003, an Israeli research group at Ben-Gurion University of the Negev compared reflex zone indications of illness with conventional medical diagnoses and found considerable correlations.

Two important studies were carried out in 2006: the effectiveness of the foot reflex zones for motor skills following a stroke was established at the Guangxi College, a university in Nanjing, China, while a study by Professor Christine Uhlemann at the University of Jena, Germany, proved the effectiveness of massage of the foot zones for complaints arising from arthrosis of the knee. Finally, a study conducted at the UK's University of Ulster in 2010 demonstrated that the foot zones could reduce pain in those suffering from multiple sclerosis. These examples only concern using the feet as a reflex zone system; there are of course corresponding proofs of effectiveness for many other reflex zones.

Reflex zone systems, such as those in the ear or skull, are often treated with needles, but this is in no way to suggest that reflex zones follow the principles of acupuncture. Taking the ears as an example, many cultures have paid special attention to the ears, but in the 1950s, French doctor Paul Nogier was the first to establish a connection between certain zones on the ear and other physical structures with his 'pinch test': he measured the skin's electrical resistance at the ear, pinched the test subject on the knee and then took another measurement from the ear. As the areas identified on the ears of the test subjects were similar, he concluded that this was where the knee point must be – a discovery that has since helped many people suffering with knee complaints. He went on to gradually work out the location of the other organs and was able to map out the ears fully.

This illustrates the principle of reflexology clearly, namely that each reflex zone is associated with a specific physical structure or an organ, whereas in acupuncture such points are gateways to a system of energy channels that cover the entire body. Depending on which of these channels has too much or too little energy, one of the gateways or acupuncture points must be 'stimulated'. Unlike with reflex zones, acupuncture points are not directly associated with an organ. Take the case of our meat feast example: to apply acupuncture, we would have to identify in each instance which channel had been disrupted and only then would we be in a position to insert needles into the appropriate gateways or to massage them with finger pressure. Unlike with reflex zones, this diagnostic procedure is a complex undertaking and a high art indeed.

Once the greater extent of the 'where' – the mapping of the zones – has been established and a variety of options for the correct treatment identified, the question of 'how' then becomes all the more important: what paths do the impulses take on their journey from, say, the gall bladder to the reflex zones and back? It should be made clear that this remains unknown – traditional nerve paths are of only limited use in such cases. There are nonetheless two possibilities that seem plausible and which probably apply in parallel. One is that the information may use the vast network of the autonomic nervous system (responsible for our largely unconscious 'fight or flight' and 'rest and digest' responses), which covers every single part of the body with a total length of approximately ten circumferences of the earth – in every one of us. The other is that there is a long-distance 'radio communications' link connecting every cell of the body.

Imagine that the autonomic network functions like the internet, with the organs using their internet access to send and receive 'emails' to and from the reflex zones; in addition to this, we have a fascinating inner 'mobile' network. In the 1970s, German biophysicist Professor Popp discovered that all our cells are connected with one another by means of ultraweak biological laser light, known as biophotons; this means that our cells have a kind of text hotline, through which they can pass on information about their condition. If it's technically possible to switch on a printer in New York from London, we should have no reason to doubt that the gall bladder is capable of sending an 'autonomic email' or a 'light text' to the relevant zones. Despite all the uncertainty surrounding how such impulses might be transported, one thing is certain: the information does arrive.

The entire Earth has now been mapped – with the last undiscovered areas having being explored during the last century – and we are now getting ready to explore space, but in so doing, we are in danger of overlooking the fact that the skin – the surface of the body – is another universe waiting to be discovered. We can only hope that interest in the reflex zones will encourage research in this direction, so that the unmapped areas on our skin will soon be a part of history, too.

Reflex zones:
One of humanity's success stories

It is likely that it all began with body painting and tattoos: 350,000-year-old pigments discovered by British scientists in Zambia suggest that our Stone Age ancestors not only immortalised hunting scenes on rock walls but also drew designs on their skin. Such rituals still exist today – from the ancient cultures of Aboriginal Australians to the San people of South Africa's Kalahari – intended to appease the gods and spirits when illness occurs. By the time rational thought began to emerge around 80,000 years ago, we already had a rich tradition of healing techniques at our disposal, and, over the thousands of years up until the present day, this knowledge has been increasingly systematised and shaped into methods and techniques. It gave rise to the first healing techniques of herbalism and targeted massage, and some points and zones in particular have clearly stood the test of time, as revealed by the tattooed marks on the skin of a man from the Chalcolithic period who came to an icy end in the Ötztal Alps that lie between Austria and Italy. Known as 'Ötzi', he provides the first evidence of a 'somatotopic' system or, put more simply, reflex zones.

Ötzi's tattoos reveal a considerable similarity to the point system used in acupuncture and show that Europeans already possessed an advanced medical culture at the time. It also allows us to conclude that reflex zones have been used as a treatment method since the dawn of Man. Examples are found in the most diverse historic cultures and eras, such as the 4,300-year-old Egyptian wall paintings in a physician's tomb in Saqqara, descriptions provided by the Chinese Wang Li 2,400 years ago and images from the Mayan culture of pre-Columbian America dating back some 1,600 years.

In the modern era, the reflex zones acted as a kind of 'godfather' at the baptism of neurology as a true science in the the 19th century.

The man who oversaw this transition was English neurologist Sir Henry Head, who described the dermatomes (the links between the stacks of spinal nerves, the organs and the zones of the skin) in 1893. Friedrich Rudolph Voltolini, a rhinologist from Breslau, had demonstrated the connection between certain zones in the nose and the female reproductive organs some ten years previously, and in 1900, at Berlin's Charité hospital, Professor Wilhelm Fliess was able to help release many women from abdominal pain by chemically cauterising these reflex zones with cocaine. Today, instead of cauterising the nasal zones with cocaine, essential oils are applied gently with cotton buds, and the zones are just as effective as they were when they were discovered more than a hundred years ago.

A further milestone in the history of reflexology was achieved when American physician William Fitzgerald decoded the system underlying the foot reflex zones; he had observed that native Americans paid particular attention to the feet and, having subsequently discovered that the feet represent a mirror image of the human body, he was able to follow up his findings by constructing a map of the body's organs on the feet. He later applied this systematic approach to the hands.

A series of reflexology pioneers appeared on the scene from around 1950, creating further maps of the surface of our bodies: Paul Nogier discovered the ear reflex zones in 1952, Anton Strobl described the zone system on the tongue in 1957, Hans Zeitler uncovered the zones of the skull in 1978 and, at the beginning of the 1980s, Rudolf Siener demonstrated that highly effective reflex zones are even to be found on the lower thighs. We now know of more than forty reflex zone systems on the surface of the body that we can get to grips with in the truest sense of the phrase.

Although the study of reflex zones has expanded considerably since the middle of the 20th century, there is still much to learn. New systems are being discovered all the time: in 1991, Toshikatsu Yamamoto described zones on the head and abdomen, and in the mid 1990s, Rita Klowersa located a reflex zone system on the collar bone; Jochen Gleditsch has referred to the 'lymph belt' and it is reasonable to suppose there are still a few more surprises left in store for us on our skin.

Since the last century, the reflex zones have enjoyed triumphant success in the field of natural healing, the effects of which are now also being felt in lay use. More and more people are beginning to realise that many day-to-day complaints can be relieved through simple massage of the reflex zones, particularly using the hands. The techniques follow a clear basic principle, are easy to use and work surprisingly well, as so many sceptics have now been forced to admit.

Following this example, other reflex zone systems are now being adopted as part of the 'first aid kit' for everyday ailments. So from the earliest humans to the present day, the story of the reflex zone systems has been one of success, of a kind achieved by only very few medical techniques.

Massage tried and trusted, a classic technique

The priest-physicians of the Pharaohs used it, the Ancient Greek physician Galen was aware of it and even Avicenna, the greatest Arabian doctor of the Middle Ages, wrote descriptions of it: we know of no culture that did not use massage; it could be one of the oldest known treatments.

Massage is used virtually everywhere and in all kinds of circumstances: we rub painful areas after a fall, physiotherapists use manual therapy to work on a joint that is not functioning properly, and the sense of touch alone works absolute wonders when a mother places her hand on a child's bruise. Given the fundamental nature of the treatment, it is not surprising that a wide range of techniques has developed, all with one thing in common: the only tools required are the hands and the goal is to improve health and wellbeing.

The effects of massage are impressive: it reduces pain, stimulates the metabolism and also harmonises the whole body. As the circulation is boosted, the supply of oxygen and nutrients to the tissues is improved, the elimination of metabolic waste products is promoted and the body's ability to self-heal is activated, relaxing and soothing the patient and bringing mental balance. Its specific effects on the internal organs and the autonomic nervous system help reflex zone massage to improve the body's inner harmony and to release pent-up energy so it can flow more freely throughout the body. As massage allows us to literally 'get in touch' and 'get to grips' with the whole person, every form of massage is ultimately a way of approaching healing for both body and soul.

Of the many massage techniques that have become established in addition to effleurage and circular stroking, 'sunray' (radiating) strokes, spiral circling and basic unblocking are particularly popular. These are all techniques that are simple and easy to use, bearing in mind that reflex zone massage should always be pleasant and should never cause pain, as indeed should be the case in order to achieve the kind of wellbeing that is expected.

Effleurage

This massage technique involves exerting slight pressure as the practitioner slides their hands over the skin. These light and superficial strokes are used when beginning a massage, to make first contact with a client and their body. Effleurage is also a suitable technique to balance basic unblocking and other techniques.

Circular stroking

This involves making slow circles with the fingers as the practitioner presses into the depths of the tissue. Here, the fingers do not slide over the skin but work within the limits of the skin's pliability. These circular strokes are used to locate specific points and for topical treatments.

Basic unblocking

Irrespective of which zone is being treated, basic unblocking remains the central technique in reflexology and involves a calm and steady lingering with no movement, applying firm but painless pressure to a reflex zone point. After around five to ten slow breaths, you will feel how your fingers actually sink into the tissue and, when the point yields in this way, the body is ready for change and for further techniques. Basic unblocking is often enough on its own to deliver some relief, but to intensify the effect while applying the technique, ask your client to imagine blowing up a beautiful balloon at the point being treated. You can then go on to treat the reflex zone with some compensatory or radiating strokes.

Radiating strokes

According to an old saying, tension begets tension but relaxation sends out ripples, and this is doubly true for massaging the reflex zones. When using radiating strokes, start from a problematic zone point and distribute the tension relief into the surrounding area by softly stroking the skin with radial 'sunray' strokes.

Whichever technique you use, always remember that massage involves using energy in a beneficial way, and it doesn't matter whether you are giving or receiving a massage – either way, it should always be pleasant and enjoyable.

Complementary techniques:
oils, stones and other tools

It may be something of a cliché that it is seasoning and spices that make a meal really tasty, but this also applies to reflexology. In addition to herbal poultices and creams, other 'ingredients' that complement massage treatments especially well are essential oils and gemstones. These should ideally be rounded off with a liberal dash of undisturbed time and some herbal tea, but, as with cooking, too many ingredients can also spoil the broth: two additional ingredients per 'reflex zone dish' constitute the best recipe for enjoyment.

First of all, however, there is one general principle in reflex zone massage that overrides all others: always keep things pleasant and never cause pain. The exceptions to this rule apply to a very few professional treatments in which needles, cupping glasses or injections are used, but these techniques are used by professional expert healers only.

Reflex zone massage with essential oils

Essential oils are an excellent accompaniment to reflex zone massage, although these refined plant essences should never be used neat – they should always be diluted, with around one part essential oil to 10–20 parts neutral oil, such as jojoba, avocado, almond or sesame. When choosing an essential oil, trust your nose and follow your instincts. If you want to be absolutely sure of your choice, try out the relevant oil using a muscle strength test. From a practical point of view, it's a good idea to make up a mixture of around 7–10 favourite oils in 20ml vials (available at pharmacies) and seal them with pipette lids.

Reflex zone massage with gemstones

Hildegard von Bingen described the healing power of gemstones and the ancient Babylonians and Romans had knowledge of it, too; it has a long history and is now undergoing a renaissance. Simple tumbled stones or crystal wands can be used for reflex zone massage, while gemstone spheres and special gemstone wands are particularly suited to reflex zone systems with a larger surface area, such as the back. All these gemstone tools harmonise the energy field and support the effects of the massage. Again, follow your instincts when selecting gemstones, opting for those that suit you best. Apply the stones carefully to the relevant reflex zones using soft, slow strokes. Gemstones, spheres and wands are available in all good crystal and mineral shops.

Herbal poultices and creams

The use of herbal poultices has a long history – steamed bags of hay flowers or herbs were traditionally placed on painful areas to ease rheumatism, lightly fried onion was wrapped in a cloth and laid on the chest for bronchitis, and creams were originally just another way of applying herbs to the skin.

To make a modern herbal poultice for reflex zones, fill a muslin bag with a tablespoon of tea herbs and steam in a sieve over boiling water for about 10 minutes. Place this lukewarm (not hot!) bag of herbs on the appropriate zone for the organ you wish to treat, cover with a warm towel and leave for about 15 minutes. Choose the herbs for the poultice according to their various healing powers – a good herbal guide is invaluable here. It is of course even simpler to use creams and oils containing herbal ingredients; simply massage into the zones, cover and leave to soak in.

The client should always drink plenty of liquids with each reflex zone treatment, preferably water or herbal tea. This tea mixture complements reflex zone therapy particularly well: 20g Acorus calamus (sweet flag), 30g angelica root, 20g speedwell, 20g mint leaves and 10g centaury. Leave to infuse in hot water for about 8–10 minutes and drink two cups a day for about three weeks. Ask a herbalist or alternative practitioner to help you adjust the balance of herbs to suit personal requirements.

Seeking and finding reflex zones

Everybody is different, even though all our bodies have the same basic design; the same is true of the reflex zones, so even the most perfect reflex zone map is just a plan of the body giving pointers as to which organs or physical structures are affected. As the with the streets and rivers on a conventional map, the points on a reflex zone map are only representative, but the more the map directs you, the more useful it is. The relevant organ zones are approximately where they are indicated on the map, so you have to feel your way to the right point. With practice your fingers will become more sensitive and you will find it increasingly easy to locate the right reflex zones. To be absolutely sure you find the right zone, make slow, circular movements with the fingers – not sliding along the skin, but just making circles as large as is feasible in the location. This will allow you to find any places that feel sensitive or tender, and these are the areas to which you should pay particular attention.

Compared to the area around it, the tissue of an unbalanced reflex zone may seem different, appearing, for example, to be more sensitive or feel softer, less firm or firmer, more tense, swollen or shrunken. The appearance of the zone may also be different and may include reddening, paleness, spots or eczema, but noting changes in how the skin looks is the limit of a layperson's skills – any actual problems with the skin itself should always be treated by an expert. A muscle strength test will give more exact results to back up your findings, but these techniques require considerable experience and are generally only used as part of professional reflex zone treatments or therapies.

Using reflex zones

The state of physical and spiritual harmony that we call 'wellbeing' cannot be manufactured from scratch, but it will come about provided the suitable basic conditions are created and the body's control centre – the autonomic nervous system (see page 11) – is involved. The autonomic regulatory system vacillates continually between actively responding to stimuli and the body's need for rest. If we have too much of the former, we say we are stressed, and too much of the latter, we feel as though we just can't quite get our brain 'into gear', but either way, our 'wellbeing' is affected.

Reflexology supports the regulation of these two inner states and helps us to maintain our autonomic pendulum in a harmonious rhythm. Regular self-treatment promotes a kind of active calmness and composure (although it's much nicer when someone else provides the treatment, of course), indicating pure wellbeing for body and soul. The reflex zones that are most suitable for this are on the hands, feet and head.

1. Hand reflex zones

This technique allows you to activate both parts of the autonomic nervous system: stroking along each finger from the tip to the wrist (working from the thumb to the little finger) should be followed with soft circular movements of the thumb across the whole surface of the palm, with basic unblocking at the sensitive points. The back of the hand is treated in the same manner, with more stroking movements to finish. Depending on the time available, a session of this kind can last between three minutes and half an hour. The same approach can also used when treating the foot reflex zones in the corresponding way.

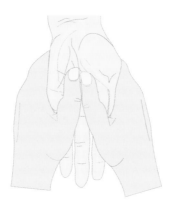

2. Skull reflex zones

The scalp contains a series of reflex zones, which play a particularly important role in the autonomic regulation of muscle tension, so it is always worth trying these massages to improve movement and coordination after a stroke. Whether using self-massage of the skull zones, or treating this area in others, massage slowly and systematically across the scalp from front to back. Take your time and don't rub; gently knead the scalp backwards and forwards on the skull.

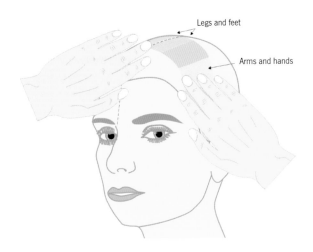

Legs and feet

Arms and hands

Complementary techniques

To achieve balance in the autonomic nervous system and wellbeing, use a mixture of essential oils uniting 'fire and ice' to massage the reflex zones of the hands and feet. Add a drop each of a stimulating oil (such as rosemary, sandalwood or ginger) and a calming oil (such as lemon balm, camomile or lavender) to around 20 drops of a neutral oil (see page 17).

Massage using the hands is perfect for the skull reflex zones. You can also massage these zones as part of your haircare routine by using a top-quality organic hair oil before washing.

This recipe for a herbal tea is based on the fire and ice principle and provides particular support for the autonomic nervous system: add boiling water to 20g each of angelica and valerian root, mint and lemon balm leaves and leave to brew for around 10 minutes. Drink daily for two to three weeks as a supplement.

The gemstones most suitable for these massages are rock crystal, bronzite and tiger eye.

Age-related ailments

As Karl Valentin, the Bavarian performer and film producer of the 1930s, pointed out, 'If you want to get old, you have to live a long time', and we now all hope to reach a great age while still retaining our physical and mental health. Scientists have identified the following as being detrimental to the body's strength and vitality in the ageing process:

Free radicals are harmful to cell structures, weakening defence against diseases of old age such as rheumatism, arteriosclerosis and Parkinson's.

Hormone deficiency with increasing age is detrimental to communication within the body.

Ageing genetic information in the chromosomes degrades the quality of newly formed cells and their functions.

A weakened immune system is linked with compromised defence against disease in old age.

Reduced metabolism arising from old age is harmful to detoxification functions.

Treatment of the reflex zones cannot halt these processes, but it can relieve many of the aches and pains that complicate life as we get older. Treating the hands, feet and ears in particular can help to improve quality of life and keep the body fit.

1. Hand and foot reflex zones

Older people often find it difficult to reach their own feet, but when these massages are applied by relatives or professionals, remarkable improvements in general wellbeing are often achieved; the reflex zones of the hands are also suitable for self-massage.

The essential massage technique for both the feet and hands consists of numerous strokes along the spinal zones towards the toes and/or fingers. You can then move on to mental stimulation by manipulating the brain zones, before finishing the treatment by massaging the entire reflex zone system with balancing strokes.

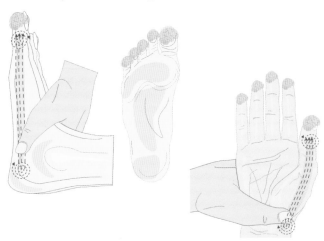

2. Ear reflex zones

To achieve inner harmony of the body, which is essential in old age, treating the reflex zones of the ears is recommended. Begin by using several firm strokes to massage the spinal zones of the earlobe from bottom to top; next, stroke along the edge of the ear in the same direction. Then, massage the brain zones by taking the earlobe between thumb and index finger and manipulating it thoroughly. To finish, carry out the strokes described above in the opposite direction.

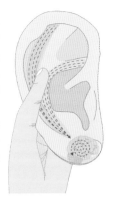

Complementary techniques

Our lifestyles can play a big part in helping us to retain our vitality. A positive attitude to life with happiness, healthy nutrition including plenty of vitamins, plenty of movement and exercise in a natural environment, and even enjoying a small glass of beer or wine (but not smoking): these are the most important things we can do to ensure the gods of healthy ageing smile down on us.

From the age of 50 onwards, it is also important to intercept free radicals: these reactive molecules or atoms rip electrons from our cell structures, while what we call free radical interceptors are substances that are able to bind to free radicals and neutralise their harmful potential. Vitamins C and E, the coenzyme Q10, flavonoids (phytochemicals found in the colourful pigments of plants) and enzymes have proved to be particularly effective. The interception of these harmful substances is ultimately one of the most promising ways of being able to exercise a positive influence on the ageing process.

Apatite, fossilised wood and haematite all have a good track record with many complaints of old age.

Backache

Around half of us experience unpleasant back pain on a daily basis, but the causes are not quite so clear as may appear at first glance; an unemployed person, for example, is considerably more at risk of suffering backache than an office worker, and a graduate has more chance of escaping a herniated intervertebral disc than someone who left school at 16.

The solutions are exactly the same for everyone, however: more exercise, less stress and proper relaxation. Fortunately, more than 90 per cent of these back complaints clear up by themselves within a few days or weeks, but quality of life is massively reduced when they strike. The enforced withdrawal from daily life that results also provides an opportunity to try and identify the root causes. As well as consulting a doctor, it means examining your lifestyle. The reflex zones can help break the downward spiral of pain–tension–more pain and accelerate a return to normality.

1. Hand reflex zones

The reflex zones of the hands can bring relief from back pain, as many sufferers have already discovered. After stroking along the spinal zones from top to bottom, explore these zones systematically and in the same direction with small circular strokes, unblocking any sensitive reflex zone points. Previous treatments have shown that the areas of maximum disturbance are those that react most energetically and require the longest amount of time to relax (but make sure the massage is always pleasant). To boost the technique, breathe directly into the point treated, and imagine you are blowing up a balloon there.

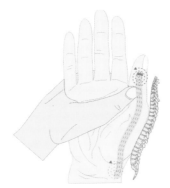

2. Ear reflex zones

This kind of treatment for back pain has a long tradition, as French doctor Paul Nogier found out when he discovered this reflex zone system in 1950. Several of his patients had small cauterisation marks on their ears where lay healers had successfully treated their backache.

The dramatic kind of treatment that would have created these marks is not required when these reflex zones are treated at home, however. Finger massage of the zones between thumb and index finger has sufficient potential to reduce pain, and in particular, if basic unblocking is repeated every hour, experience has shown that relief will come swiftly.

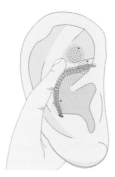

Complementary techniques

The main aim with all back complaints is to stabilise the entire spinal column by balancing the muscles of the back in a way that will provide lasting relief, along with strengthening the muscles of the stomach. Once this equilibrium has been restored, the back will recover. This is when a physiotherapist should be consulted. Relaxation is also a part of establishing this balance. Autogenic training or meditation can be of help, too. One contributing factor that is often underestimated is smoking. Experts have labelled it 'smoker's lumbar disc', as smokers have an increased risk of developing chronic back pain problems.

The following essential oils are suitable as a complement to reflex zone massage and for rubbing into the back: bergamot, dill, sandalwood, frankincense, marjoram and rosemary. Tumbled gemstones of rock crystal, tiger eye and rhodonite are especially helpful for massage or placing on the body.

Bladder weakness

Cold feet, infections, mental tension and prostate or womb conditions are the most common causes of bladder problems.

People suffering from these know the symptoms only too well: the pressure makes it feel like the bladder is completely full, but only a negligible amount of liquid is actually passed, and they feel especially drained physically and mentally, and lacking in vitality and vigour.

Looking at the background to these problems, they generally seem to crop up when we feel particularly tense or exhausted. The sphincter that normally keeps the bladder tightly closed has to be opened actively and if the sufferer is feeling especially tense or the sphincter is weak, the ability to control it is disrupted. As bladder function is subject to autonomic control, however, the reflex zones can provide good support; they will not remove the causes of the problem, but they can soothe an irritable bladder and relieve the accompanying symptoms.

1. Foot reflex zones

Treating the reflex zones of the feet is a promising way of relieving bladder problems. The sacral nerves, part of the autonomic nervous system responsible for controlling functions in the lower abdomen, can also be influenced from the bladder reflex zone area. The principal massage technique consists of relaxing circular movements in the bladder zones. Interspersed with these, basic unblocking at the sensitive reflex

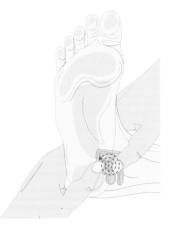

zone points may also be carried out, finishing with effleurage of the surrounding area and completing the foot treatment with balancing strokes.

2. Back reflex zones

The massage of connective tissue is a professional treatment for the back zones and results in better autonomic regulation of the internal organs. This can also be achieved with self-treatment. Although only a few of the reflex zone areas of the back are reachable, the bladder is one of these. To carry out self-massage, lean forward slightly and place your fingers to either side of the top of the intergluteal cleft (at the top of the buttocks). From here, move outwards across this reflex zone area, making vigorous circular strokes, and follow with radiating strokes in all directions from the reflex points. To finish, place your hands on the skin and take a few breaths to relax.

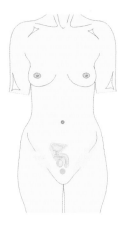 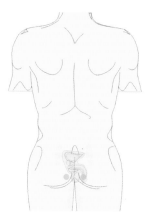

Reflex zone massage allows you to influence the whole area around a sensitive reflex zone point, one consequence being that the organ is stimulated and its function normalised. For this reason, a pressing need to pass water after treatment is often felt, which is linked to an activation of the metabolism and the connective tissue surrounding the organ. The treatment allows access to the controls of the autonomic nervous system and therefore the interaction between the organs.

With bladder complaints in particular, it is important to drink plenty of fluids, preferably water or tea. This herbal drink is good for the bladder: take 30g stinging nettle leaves, 20g goldenrod leaves, 30g dandelion root and 20g bearberry leaves and leave them to brew in hot water for about 10–12 minutes. Drink three cups daily as a course of treatment over three weeks.

If you would like to use oils, sandalwood is especially suitable as a complement to reflex zone massage, while in terms of gemstones, aventurine and dumortierite are recommended, either as tumbled stones or wands.

Colds

You have tried so hard to stay cold-free but unfortunately it hasn't worked: your throat is sore, you want to cough, your nose is now blocked and you feel run down. You have caught a cold. Your immune system was obviously in a weakened state and not up to withstanding a viral invasion. A weakened immune system is not an illness as such, but it makes you more vulnerable to becoming ill. Stress, cold feet, wet weather, draughts, overtiredness or just circumstances – things in life that are getting you down – are likely to be the culprits. The ways of coping with a cold have been tried and tested for generations: cough sweets, vitamin C, hot lemon and home or over-the-counter remedies from the chemist. In addition to these, the reflex zones of the hands and feet can help to relieve the symptoms that are making you suffer, but most importantly, your immune system needs some peace and quiet to see off the virus.

1. Hand reflex zones

Left untreated, an average cold lasts around eight days; with treatment, a week! In other words, you just have to wait for it to take its course, even reflex zones won't alter that. But they can help when you have nothing at hand to ease the symptoms. This simple technique helps to relieve a sore throat: place the fingertips of one hand in the 'webs' between the fingers of the other and massage them this way about 7–10 times, repeating the procedure once or twice every hour. To finish, interlace the fingers of both hands and then pull them apart slowly, exerting mild pressure. You will nearly always feel a slight improvement in symptoms afterwards.

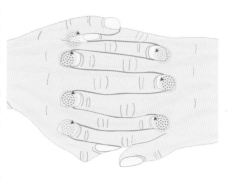

2. Foot reflex zones

A cold is on the whole harmless if accompanied only by mild fever and it doesn't last longer than a week. Cold, chilly feet aggravate a cold, whereas warm feet help to boost the immune system, which is why massaging the feet is helpful in alleviating a cold.

After bathing the feet in warm water, indulge them and stroke and

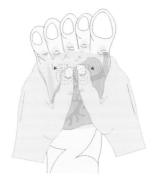

knead each foot in turn. If any zones feel tender and sensitive, soothe them with basic unblocking, before finishing with more strokes; if you can find someone to do this treatment for you, it is even more pleasant of course.

Complementary techniques

If you catch a cold, there is a wide range of home remedies available that should always be tried first. Antibiotics are often prescribed far too early – they do nothing to combat viruses and are only really appropriate if the viral infection is compounded by a bacterial one.

Until you reach that point, you can safely rely on home remedies, such as inhaling decongestants, rubs for the back and chest, warm foot baths with salt, herbal teas and homeopathic medicines. Essential oils are perfect for inhaling and can also be used for body rubs: pine needle, camomile and lavender are all suitable oils (but always use them in dilution).

This healing herbal tea recipe relieves colds: 30g marshmallow root, 20g sage, 10g thyme, 10g lime blossom and 10g elderflower blossom (leave to brew in hot water for 10 minutes, drink two or three cups daily). The primary aim is of course to strengthen the body's defences over the long term so you are ready to face the next wave of cold germs. Gemstones to boost the immune system include heliotrope and ocean agate.

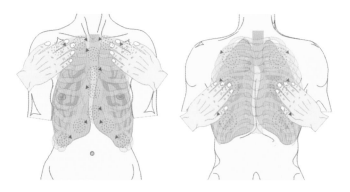

Cold feet

As well as being extremely unpleasant, cold feet can lead to bladder irritation, abdominal complaints, haemorrhoids or colds, to name just a few of the problems associated with them. Unfortunately for smokers, this habit is also a major culprit, causing serious circulatory problems and smokers with cold feet are at high risk of developing 'smoker's leg'.

Whether your feet are warm or cold depends on your circulation, which in turn is determined by the regulation of the blood flow through the small arteries. There are a number of ways that this can be improved – washing with cold water, as recommended by the German naturopath Father Kneipp, is just as effective as plenty of walking, playing sport or sessions in the sauna. But what can you do when your feet start to get cold sitting in the cinema, or in a garden in summer, for example? This is where the reflex zones of the skull and ear can step in, helping your feet to warm up from the inside within minutes.

1. Skull reflex zones

These reflex zones allow you to access muscle coordination, proprioception and the circulation of the musculoskeletal systems. The zones relating to blood vessel control in the feet are easy to find: following a line up the centre of the face from the nose, the correct points are to the immediate right and left of a spot on this line about three fingers' width above the hairline. These reflex zone points, which often feel softer and more sensitive than the surrounding area, can be massaged extensively but gently using circular finger movements (you may need to use a tumbled stone of snowflake obsidian as well). A feeling of warmth will spread through the feet after a few minutes.

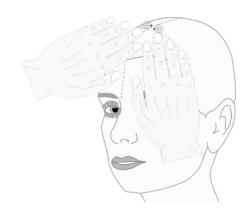

2. Ear reflex zones

The foot and leg zones are also found on the ears and can be used to improve circulation. These reflex zones are located in an easily identifiable triangle in the ear and can be massaged firmly. Circular strokes are best used in this instance. Pinch these zones on both ears at the same time, holding them between thumb and index finger. Hold them for seven to ten breaths, which should be enough to make the feet feel

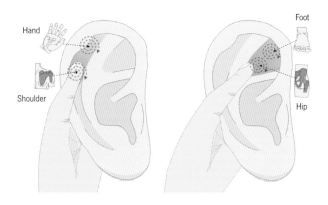

warmer. Both this technique and that described for the skull have also proved effective for treating sore limbs or muscles that have been over-exerted hiking or playing sport.

Complementary techniques

Feet need to be well looked after, but in the case of cold feet, not in the literal sense – simply taking care of the feet themselves – but in a broader sense, by looking after the blood vessels and circulation. A topical treatment is to massage them with a soothing foot balm that promotes circulation. Most shop-bought foot creams are enriched with essential oils, but you can also treat your feet regularly with your own mixture of oils: those containing rosemary, sandal-wood, bergamot or frankincense oil are especially beneficial.

Snowflake obsidian is an ideal gemstone for skull reflex zone massage, either in the form of a wand or as a tumbled stone. When used as a palm stone, snowflake obsidian can also help the hands to warm up.

The best way to keep your circulatory system in good condition is of course to walk or hike regularly, or to do Nordic walking or some other physical activity, which will help to maintain healthy functioning blood vessels and ensure the core of the body's warmth extends to the feet.

Coping with stress

Taking a little time out has become difficult in the modern world – the desire for relaxation is challenged by the increasing demands of our professional and private lives – and yet we still hope to be able to switch off. Even if we do manage to find a moment of peace, however, we find our thoughts still running on and on and round and round, like a hamster on a wheel. Massaging the reflex zones is of course not sufficient in cases of extreme stress, when a doctor should be consulted, or a relaxation technique practised, such as autogenic training or Jacobson's progressive muscle relaxation technique or, if none of these bring relief, medication should be prescribed. When faced with minor symptoms of stress, however, the reflex zones are an invaluable aid to halting the hamster wheel and escaping the downward spiral into deeper stress.

The reflex zones of the feet, hands and face in particular have proved effective in turning things around and promoting relaxation.

While treating the zones of the feet will enable you to switch off at the end of a stressful day, those on the hands can be used as an emergency measure during a stressful day, and the facial zones work well for deep relaxation at a beauty salon or a wellness spa.

1. Foot reflex zones

Massaging the two centres at the upper and lower ends of the spinal column can significantly reduce the potential for stress. To begin, stroke the sides of both feet 5–7 times, working from the big toe down to the heel, breathing out slowly with each stroke. Cover the same area with slow circular strokes before moving on to basic unblocking of the sensitive points at the big toe joint and at the bottom around the inside of the ankle. Finish with further effleurage of the link between the top and bottom of the foot. The points and the technique are the same for the hand reflex zones.

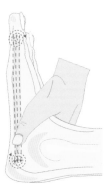

2. Facial reflex zones

Beauticians and their clients know just how relaxing and 'stress-busting' a facial massage can be. The reflex zones help to get the 'emotional juices' flowing in every organ and to supply the energy they need. A break in a meeting at work is a good opportunity for a quick facial reflex zone massage – use soft, circular movements to get the skin and facial muscles moving. The effect is amazing, especially when you return relaxed from the break while others are still stressed. The nicest option is, of course, a complete professional reflex zone facial massage.

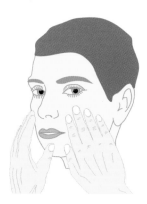

Complementary techniques

Whether you're centering yourself in preparation for a meeting or enjoying a leisurely relaxation session, stress reduction should always have some kind of framework. You might be able to set aside a fairly generous window of time for the treatment and to give yourself the space to enjoy it, although just concentrating on a few breaths in and out before a business meeting will often be enough to do the trick. In both cases, however, you will be in a position to recharge your 'mental batteries' more swiftly.

A lavender pillow is also a tried-and-trusted way to de-stress at night. All that's needed is some dried lavender from the herbalist's, which can be tied up in a little cotton bag and placed under the pillow. Along with discouraging unnecessary thoughts while deepening sleep, it has the added advantage of fending off mosquitoes. Lavender oil is also suitable for reflex zone massage.

A tumbled stone or crystal wand made from black tourmaline, tiger eye or bronzite can be carried as a touchstone or used for massage to combat the effects of stress.

Digestive problems

'Death sits in the gut', as Austrian physician Dr F.X. Mayr said at the start of the 20th century, and much of our wellbeing is dependent on a good digestive system, especially health and happiness; even the language that we use hints at this connection: we talk of something being 'stomach-churning', or 'to have a bellyful of something', or perhaps we have a feeling 'in our gut' that something is going to 'go down the toilet'.

The large intestine is responsible for eliminating waste products and faeces, but additionally functions as a window on our psyches if we are unable to digest something either physically or mentally. The reflex zones of the large intestine located on the face are of special significance and skin blemishes often appear in the area around the chin. Unfortunately, direct treatment of these zones has no notable effect, but they are stimulated during a cosmetic face massage. However, treatment of the foot and tongue reflex zones allows us to exert a much greater influence on the digestive functions of both body and mind, and to achieve outcomes that will lift a great burden from us in the most literal of senses.

1. Tongue reflex zones

It's hard to believe that this muscle in the mouth is also a reflex zone system, but it is the case and it as has been known in Ayurvedic medicine for more than 3,000 years: the tongue is a mirror of the entire digestive system. As part of their daily purification ritual, people living in India use a tongue scraper, to remove tongue deposits, but also as an effective reflex zone treatment to stimulate the digestion. In the event of digestive problems, the technique can also be applied by using a second toothbrush or a tongue scraper to gently massage the upper part of the tongue after cleaning the teeth in the morning.

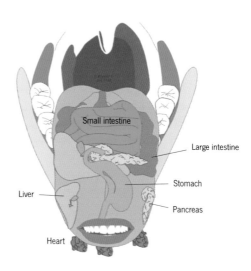

2. Foot reflex zones

These reflex zone techniques are extremely effective for digestive problems, although you may experience an urgent need to pass water afterwards and bowel movements are often more frequent later the same or on the following day.

The ideal technique for this kind of massage involves gentle but firm circular strokes, complemented with basic unblocking of any sensitive points, followed by radiating strokes. In the case of longer-lasting digestive problems, beginning with two treatments per week and then repeating them at intervals of two weeks is recommended.

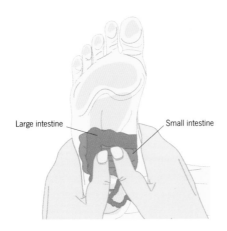

Large intestine | Small intestine

Complementary techniques

Digestive problems are generally the result of a number of years of poor diet, often combined with a lack of exercise. So it is wise to take advantage of these treatments and also to use them as the impetus to change to a high-fibre, wholefood diet. Avoid using laxatives, as they can be addictive and bowel movement comes to rely on them, but instead try to train the bowels to empty at the same time every day.

One of the most important things for the bowels is exercise: the inner muscles of the hip, which lift the leg forwards when you take a step, massage the bowel as you walk or run, supporting its proper function, activating the metabolism and burning calories. Drinking a digestive tea is a helpful complement to this; the tea's aromatic, bitter compounds will stimulate bowel movements and detoxify the intestines: try 30g angelica root, 20g Acorus calamus (sweet flag), 10g centaury, 20g mint leaves and 10g mugwort (leave to infuse in hot water for about 8 minutes and drink one cup daily for around two weeks).

Eye strain

Long periods of time spent sitting in front of a screen are hard on the eyes, as people who work on computers are only too well aware: your eyes start to burn, your concentration lapses and, by evening, you can't 'see straight' any more. Once you have checked with a doctor that there is nothing wrong, you come to the conclusion that you probably have a case of classic eye strain. There are usually not enough hours in the day to allow your eyes to refocus sufficient times or to give them the rest that they need and medical experts advise, and your next holiday is not yet on the horizon!

The reflex zones offer three different options for speedy relief. The first of these, the zones of the ear, was used by seafarers and artisans in the Middle Ages, the second employs the zones of the forehead and the third makes use of the reflex zones of the hand.

1. Ear reflex zones

Centuries ago, artisans working on the con-struction of cathedrals were given an earring to wear in the eye point of their left ear when their apprenticeship was finished, to improve their intuitive sight. This point (on both ears) is still effective for strengthening and relieving the eyes. For this massage, take both earlobes bet-ween thumb and index finger and rub each one well, before stroking up to the part of the ear called the antihelix and beyond to the channel behind it. Finish by making soft circles in the same direction to balance out these strokes across the whole ear, and you'll be fresh for your next task.

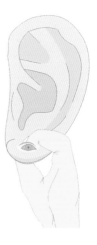

2. Forehead reflex zones

Massage of this reflex zone system, which was discovered by Toshikatsu Yamamoto, a Japanese doctor, in 1970, helps strengthen the eyes and give tired eyes a little break.

This massage is both effective and extremely pleasant. The reflex zone points are located where an imaginary line drawn up from the inner corner of the eye meets the hairline. The best treatment is to apply numerous slow circles to these points and the surrounding area, always moving the skin across the skull but without rubbing. Close your eyes during the treatment and you will enjoy it all the more.

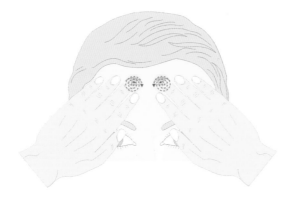

Complementary techniques

Eyebright – the name of this herb says it all. Its botanical name is Euphrasia. It is available as homeopathic pillules and you can make a herbal brew that is suitable for lukewarm compresses.

For homeopathic treatment of eye strain, Euphrasia officinalis 4x is recommended in the evening (allow five pillules to dissolve under the tongue) and use cotton wool pads soaked in lukewarm herbal tea to make eyebright compresses; leave on the eyes for around 10–15 minutes. Lavender oil and rose oil are a good complement to reflex zone massage (especially of the hands), while in terms of gemstones, rock crystal, agate and aquamarine can be beneficial for tired eyes; they help the eyes to regenerate when used for forehead massage or when worn as a decorative pendant.

The best way to look after the eyes is to rest them frequently and to change their focus by looking away from the screen into the world outside.

Fear of flying

Taking a flight can be healthy! Whether you're flying to New York on business, when you use the time to prepare some work, or are taking a holiday on the Canary Islands, when you can relax and enjoy an interesting conversation, you can still spare a few minutes for your health, even on a short flight to the Balearics. For many people, however, the trip to the airport is always accompanied by the fear of flying, but fortunately there are a number of reflex zone techniques for the hand that help ease all kinds of nervousness. These techniques have proved to be effective against stage fright and exam stress as well as fear of flying.

Travellers on long-haul flights have an additional concern to contend with: sitting for too long in the same position at great altitude increases the chances of thrombosis. However, a series of small massages of the back reflex zones – which saved the physiotherapist Elisabeth Dicke's leg back in 1928 – are a good way to prevent thrombosis during a flight. These techniques can also be used quite easily, even in the most confined spaces.

1. Hand reflex zones to fight fear of flying
This simple treatment can be highly effective in combating fear, allowing you to access the reflex zones of the brain stem, where the centre of breathing and the major autonomic control centres are located.

To begin, take the top joint of the thumb between the thumb and index finger of the other hand and roll the thumb tip in circles into the joint for about a minute. Then maintain a constant but pleasant pressure on the brain stem point just above the joint for about five to seven breaths, before finishing by rolling the thumb tip into the joint ten more times. Then swap hands. This small exercise is relaxing and will have a calming effect on the nerves for some time.

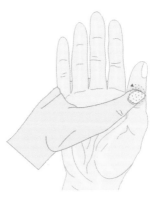

2. Back reflex zones as a means to prevent thrombosis

This simple technique can also be used on a plane: lean forward slightly in your seat and reach behind you, placing your hands so that the thumbs are lying on the iliac crests (hip bone) and the fingers are on the sacrum. Making circles with your fingers on the sacrum, slowly progress

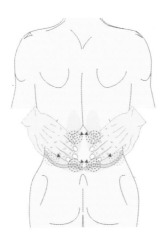

from the middle to the outside along the hip bone and back again, before repeating the process a little higher up, always massaging with your fingers. Pleasant waves of feeling will soon be felt in the back and may even reach the feet. Heighten the effect by breathing in as you touch the areas to be massaged.

Complementary techniques

If travelling with a partner, massaging each other's hand reflex zones is a great way to start a vacation as it promotes relaxation. Even though essential oils cannot generally be used on a plane to ease a fear of flying, you can take some gemstones with you: a small tumbled stone of dumortierite carried in a pocket, or with a hole drilled through it and worn as jewellery, will be of great help. Known as the 'take it easy' gemstone, it bolsters confidence in tricky situations and generally helps you to take life less seriously.

Some people experience nausea on flights; to combat this try chewing crystallized ginger, which can also be used to alleviate seasickness. Magnesite promotes relaxation and relieves cramps; it is especially effective for the legs and the heart, so always have some to hand on a flight. Both stones are inexpensive and available as pendants from good gemstone shops.

Head colds

A-choo! It's a sound that heralds a case of the sniffles. But there's no need to worry too much – you know that colds are harmless and will go in six days: two days to develop, two days in 'full flow' and two days to be on the mend. After an initial tickly feeling, your nose begins to run and one of the many cold viruses that are around has overcome your defence barriers, settled down in the mucous membranes and flooded throughout body. The membranes swell up, your nose is blocked and you feel under the weather. Antibiotics are no use; the only option is to take remedies that strengthen the immune system, homeopathy and vitamins. In the meantime, your immune system will be rustling up reinforcements and will be getting ready to stage a successful defensive battle. It will be busy renewing cells and disposing of those that have become casualties of the virus; you can provide support for this clean-up operation by drinking plenty of liquids. The swelling in the mucous membrane will ultimately go down, and massage of the reflex zones will help keep your nose and head clear.

1. Hand reflex zones

Reflex zone massage of the hand will enable you to keep a clear head when you have a cold and help keep the membranes of the whole naso-pharyngeal area open to breathe. Crucially, these techniques can be used anywhere at any time. The most important zones for this are located on the inside of the hand, between the thumb and index finger – use gentle circular strokes to massage everywhere along these areas once or twice daily and to unblock the most active reflex zone points. Between these massages, you can also gently 'milk' the 'webs' between the fingers every hour to improve lymph drainage.

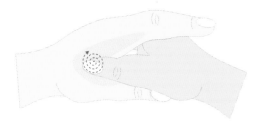

2. Ear reflex zones

The effectiveness of the reflex zones of the ear is often underestimated. A technique applied to the ear can clear a stuffy nose with surprising speed, for example, and not just when you have the sniffles. It will make it easier to breathe through the nose even when an allergy has caused the congestion and the feeling of being 'bunged up' rather than a cold – although it should be mentioned that the effects generally only last around 10–15 minutes. The bad news is that reflex zones are powerless against viruses, but the good news is that there is a technique to ease their effects that can be repeated as much as you like: all you need to do is gently massage the tragus in front of the ear canal, squeezing it as you would for basic unblocking. You will notice the treatment taking effect within about 20–30 seconds.

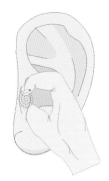

Complementary techniques

Viruses always affect the whole body and even though each strain of virus targets a different organ, the body's defensive system has to fight them on all fronts. For this reason, herbal teas (see 'Colds', page 31) act both locally and via the control centres of the immune system in the gut. The body's defence cells need substances to help them in the immune system's fight, which include vitamins C and E, enzymes and zinc.

Topical treatments for a runny nose are intended to reduce swelling in the mucous membranes, and a whole range of homeopathic nose drops and sprays is available, so products with ingredients that constrict the blood vessels can be avoided, especially as they can be addictive. It's often enough to moisten the nose with a cooking salt solution or a steam bath. Camomile, pine needle and lavender oil are all suitable for steam inhalation and for reflex zone massage. The most effective gemstones for a runny nose include heliotrope, chalcedony and fluorite.

Headaches

The head is prone to different problems – from throbbing temples with the sensation of being trapped in a vice, while a jackhammer is busy at work in the background, to having a brain that feels as though it is made of cotton wool. Fortunately, however, most of these nasty sensations go away on their own. The symptoms are as varied as the causes that may underlie them: a stiff neck, problems with the spine, metabolic disturbances, allergies, medicine, unstable blood pressure, too much stress, long periods spent sitting at the computer and much more. Essentially, any organ in the body can have a detrimental effect on the head.

Most people suffering from a headache just think of reaching for the usual analgesics, but these medicines are often also bad for the head; until the cause has been identified, you are better off using remedies that cause no side effects instead. These include reflex zone massage, which generally works just as quickly as the usual headache pills.

1. Neck reflex zones

A typical place to treat a tension headache is the neck. It seems the natural place to reduce the muscle tension that causes it, even with no knowledge of the reflex zones. Important control centres for many of the functions of the head and sensory organs are also located here, just beneath the point where the muscles of the spine meet the muscles of the neck.

For this technique, take the back of your head in your hands, with your fingers to the sides and your thumbs in the middle. From this position, make circular strokes with both thumbs to massage the central area gently but thoroughly. After basic unblocking of the maximum release_points, finish with effleurage from a line down the back of the neck out to the sides.

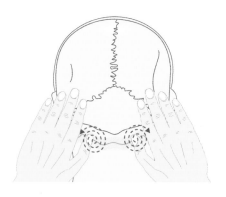

2. Hand reflex zones

Headaches are annoying and unpleasant – they can stop us from thinking clearly and be impossible to shake off. Two areas of the hand reflex zones may be of some help: the brain stem zones on the joint of the thumb enable you to influence the nerve supply to the head, while the reflex zones of the brain are in the pads of the fingers.

Basic unblocking has proved effective for the brain stem zones and, even when used on its own, can often make a situation more bearable. Rubbing the pads of the fingers together gently for a few minutes may often produce results, making a nagging stress pain disappear, or at least be eased considerably.

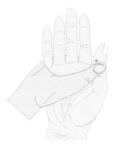

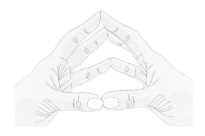

For recurrent headaches, it's also worth considering the impact of any possible mental strain in addition to any medical considerations. The expressions 'racking my brains' and the need to 'get my head round something' hint at this type of underlying cause and some honest self-appraisal may be required to pinpoint where a conflict of this kind may be proving too stressful and burdensome. Essential oils that have a beneficial effect on headaches include lemon balm, cardamom and ginger (give them a try), while the gemstones amethyst, dumortierite (the 'take it easy' stone) and garnet have also demonstrated that they work particularly well.

Ancient Indian medicine teaches the use of meditative finger positions (known as *mudras*) for many problems. One such *mudra* is also extremely effective against headaches. Using light pressure, just press the fingers of both hands together for 1–3 minutes and breathe deeply in and out over the joined fingers.

Long car journeys

You're driving your car and you feel an unpleasant tension in the back of your neck, despite the fact that the journey so far has been calm and not at all stressful. Most drivers have experienced this. However, regardless of how smooth the drive has been in terms of mental stress, it is quite another matter for the body: in a constant sitting position, with muscles tensed in anticipation, the spine has to deal with acceleration, braking manoeuvres and bends and bumps in the road. This results in a punishing workload for the cervical spine in particular, as it has to keep the head balanced throughout. If we add to the mix any stressful situations caused by driving manoeuvres, the whole body tenses up. The best solution is to take regular breaks, but unfortunately, even though the car may have been serviced and the tank filled up, on longer journeys our own 'physical vehicle' is often neglected shamefully.

Reflex zones can offer some relief here: two massage techniques – one at the base of the neck and one on the hand reflex zones – will help to reduce neck tension significantly (although obviously, using these techniques while the vehicle is in motion is strictly forbidden!).

1. Neck reflex zones

These zones are familiar from our own daily experience – when we're tense, we instinctively massage the zones at the base of the skull – but since around 1950, it has also been known that the neck line enables us to exert an influence on the cervical spine, something of which, unfortunately, not that many experts are aware.

This technique is easy to apply in a traffic jam or when you are taking a coffee break: hold your head in your hands like a ball, making gentle circular strokes from the middle to the sides and back again. Make a basic unblocking of the sensitive points and to finish, perform effleurage along the neck line from the middle to the sides.

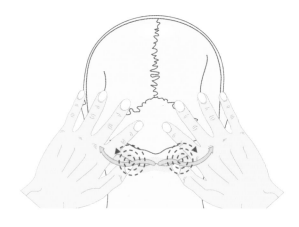

2. Hand reflex zones

Make use of the hand reflex zones whenever painful tension needs to be relieved, such as during breaks from driving.

Begin with soft circular strokes with the thumb of the opposite hand, pushing deep into the ball of the thumb. Follow this by working through the base joints of the fingers, where the reflex zones will relax the muscles of the shoulder. Impulses to reduce tension in the muscles of the neck can then be transmitted via the inner edge of the thumb; to achieve this, massage these zones from top to bottom, using light circular strokes while also devoting basic unblocking to any sensitive points.

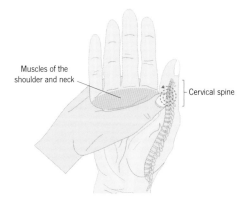

Muscles of the shoulder and neck

Cervical spine

Complementary techniques

The best way to relieve tension in the shoulder and neck region when driving is to use an ergonomic seat and take sufficient breaks, making sure to get out and stretch your legs as much as possible. Lorry drivers and travelling sales-men who cover more than 40,000km (25,000 miles) per year are particularly vulnerable to back problems and lumbago – joining a gym with the services of a physiotherapist is one way to help to prevent this.

Another alternative is to keep a tumbled stone or gemstone wand made of rock crystal, bronzite or magnesite with you when driving. Carried in the pocket or worn as a pendant, these gemstones are worthwhile complements to reflex zone massage.

For those who drive for a living, the reflex zones of the back can also be used (as described in 'Fear of flying', page 44), since a constant sitting position can often cause circulatory problems in the legs. But preventing these kinds of problems is not just a matter of getting plenty of exercise, it also involves eating a balanced diet with plenty of vital nutrients.

Men's health

A quick glance around a doctor's waiting room might lead you to think that the male sex is the healthier of the two, but unfortunately it is not the case. Men just pay a little less attention to themselves than women where illness is concerned, although men are considerably less risk-averse and more prone to accidents, suffer greater injuries and are more at risk from heart attack or stroke. Many men also suffer from enlargement of the prostate during the male menopause; in most cases it is not painful, but a permanent desire to urinate is intrusive and highly unpleasant, and when water is finally passed, it is only a small amount and brings no particular relief. It may also be compounded by the nagging fear that a man cannot perform so well sexually and 'erectile dysfunction' is a powerful drain on male self-confidence.

Unfortunately, the predilection for taking risks and sexual potency cannot be influenced via the reflex zones, but the zones on the nose and hand have proved useful for easing the symptoms that accompany prostate complaints.

1. Nose reflex zones
The nose and the reproductive organs both possess erectile tissue, although this discovery was not exploited for therapeutic purposes until 1900.

Many years earlier, in India, these zones were used to promote procreative ability by 'piercing' the side of the nose, so it is no surprise to learn that reflex zone massage of these zones normalises hormonal and sexual function.

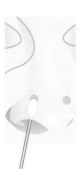

To use this technique, take a cotton bud dipped in a mixture of oils (10 parts mallow to 1 part sandalwood) and gently massage the inside of each nostril thoroughly for around 1–2 minutes. If you should experience any unpleasantness or pain, stop the massage immediately.

2. Hand and foot reflex zones

The reflex zones of the prostate can be accessed equally via the hands or feet. Reflex zone massage of the feet is suitable as a balancing technique in the evening, stimulating a complete change of mood, while the zones on the hand can be a godsend during the day.

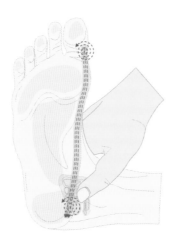

The abdominal zones are located at the base of the hands and feet, near the wrists and ankles. While a full reflex zone massage of every part of the feet should always precede targeted basic unblocking of the maximum release points, this technique can be used on the hands as required, before finishing with effleurage using circular strokes.

Complementary techniques

Men go through a menopause as well as women. From about the age of 50 or 60, many men find the prostate – a chestnut-sized organ in the lower abdomen – will become enlarged, the very latest stage at which a medical check-up examination is recommended. The precautions required to keep the prostate in trim are not limited to the lower abdomen: plenty of exercise, not too much sitting around, a low-fat diet, reduced consumption of alcohol, plenty of fluids, sexual activity and an increased intake of vitamins and zinc to intercept free radicals are also recommended. Herbal remedies that prove effective include those made with stinging nettle roots, pumpkin seeds, saw palmetto fruit and rye pollen. The essential oils that can be used for reflex zone massage are sandalwood and clary sage. Ruby zoisite, thulite, red jasper and garnet are the gemstones that influence male hormones. Whether the libido remains strong is then generally a matter for our largest sex organ, located between the ears rather than the legs!

Sensitivity to the weather

Do you have an internal barometer that helps you predict a change in the weather? Unfortunately, these weather-predicting signs can often be rather unpleasant: a scar might begin to ache, the joints stiffen up and it feels as though an ants' nest has taken up residence in your head. Animals have very finely tuned reactions to changes in the weather – frogs are famously said to croak more loudly when bad weather is brewing and humans have a similar reaction: the electrical resistance of our bodies changes when we stand over a source of running water, something that water diviners with their rods have experienced for centuries. These sensitivities increase as we get older, but unfortunately so do the complaints they cause; the most common way of tackling them is to suppress the symptoms with painkillers or just to wait until the weather changes. But the reflex zones can do better than that as they can influence what is going on in the body via the autonomic nervous system.

1. Ear reflex zones

Reflex zone massage via the autonomic nervous system can help to keep

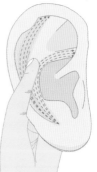

a lid on the worst of those complaints caused by changes in the weather. Dr Paul Nogier discovered the 'autonomic fold' in a channel (known as the scapha) running along the edge of the ear inside the helix (the outer edge of the ear). The spinal zones in the ear are a source of additional relief when using this technique. Begin with plenty of strokes with the thumb along the spinal zones of the earlobe, starting from the bottom (about five repetitions), and then use the same technique from bottom to top along the autonomic fold. These techniques work best when repeated every hour on those days when the problem or complaint flares up.

2. Foot reflex zones

Treating the feet to a soothing reflex zone massage in the evening will help change your mood if you are feeling a little under the weather. The most effective zones in this respect are those corresponding to three control centres of the autonomic nervous system: the reflex zones of the solar plexus, brain stem and sacrum. Begin by carrying out a general massage of the feet (with plenty of strokes down towards the heel, along the spinal zones) before treating the reflex zones of the above-mentioned control centres with basic unblocking. The treatment finishes with more effleurage, which usually elicits a feeling of cosy relaxation.

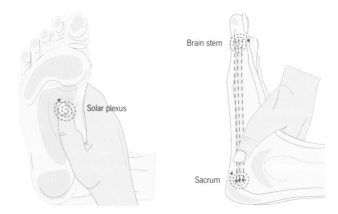

Complementary techniques

One important factor to consider with sensitivity to the weather is the presence of anything that may cause interference or an energy blockage. It could be a scar, for example, although chronic inflammation of some sort, such as a purulent tooth abscess, may also often be the culprit. The immediate living and sleeping environment should also be checked for other disruptive factors, particularly any metabolic disturbance caused by sprayed fruit and vegetables, toxins in the living space or interference from earth radiation. Exposure to these for any length of time is bad for the metabolism, which becomes less resilient as a result, provoking swifter reactions to changes in the weather. It is therefore very important to identify and eliminate any internal or external interference and, while the reflex zones cannot get rid of this entirely, they can often bring some relief. Anything that takes the pressure off the metabolism is a suitable complement to the reflex zone treatment; tea can be taken for rheumatism for example, after massaging the reflex zones with rosemary oil and frankincense oil (always diluted).

Staying alert

There are times when relaxation is not the order of the day and instead, what we really need are alertness and clarity. A splash of cold water on the face is certainly one way of achieving this, although a supply of cold water is not always available, but this is where the reflex zones can step in. The magic word here is stress – not the kind of stress that wears you down but eustress (stress that does the body good), or a positive challenge. This is where we can make use of the body's responses to stress that prepare us for fight or flight. In this state of alertness, the body's energy reserves are activated and we can access ideas and impulses more quickly.

The reflex zones provide us with a way of increasing our eustress levels in a controlled manner. The simplest technique uses the ears, while another, slightly more involved, method, uses the zones in the nose. The advantage is that the reflex zones never allow things to tip over into the kind of stress that is detrimental to us.

1. Ear reflex zones

These simple and yet highly effective ear techniques allow you to access the reflex zones of the spine and autonomic nervous system and stimulate them into activity.

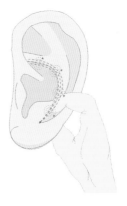

Grip both ears simultaneously between thumb and index finger, exerting firm pressure and stroking the antihelix and the channel behind it from the upper inner side down to the earlobe. Focus on maintaining a constant yet pleasant pressure. Then use the same finger position to make circles along all these ear zones. To finish, you can also gently squeeze each part of the earlobe. You will then be ready to carry on your day feeling refreshed.

2. Nose reflex zones

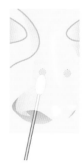

The reflex zones inside the nose are effective against headaches and are also useful for stimulating ideas. This is a rather different form of reflex zone massage: take an ordinary cotton bud, dip it in mallow oil (available from a herbalist) and use it to softly massage the inside of each nostril in gentle circles for around 1–2 minutes. This is a sensitive area so take special care and avoid any kind of unpleasant sensation. If anything feels disagreeable during the massage, stop at once. However, the treatment usually produces a really good mood, stimulating both mind and spirit.

Complementary techniques

Feelings of tiredness are a natural reaction, signalling the need to rest, but if the message is ignored, exhaustion may soon follow. When tiredness begins to set in, the reflex zones can be used to fight it, but the worse it gets, the lower the chances of success, in which case, this really is the time to rest.

Essential oils have long proved their worth as a complement to boosting vitality (used either neat in a diffuser or diluted 1:20 for massage). When activating the reflex zones of the ear, ginger, mint and sandalwood oil are particularly good. For reflex massage of the nose, use only mild oils such as rose, lemon balm or Roman camomile. Two gemstones can help you to feel more alert – heliotrope and tiger eye. Worn on the body separately or, best of all, together, they will boost your energy reserves for whatever tasks you have to do.

Stomach problems

Once upon a time it was a surfeit of fine food for kings and queens and a starvation diet for the common folk that caused stomach problems, but nowadays our digestive systems are ruined, even as children, by kebabs, burgers, hot dogs and all kinds of sugary rubbish. With the pressures of time demanding that food is eaten as quickly as possible, we often don't feel full. So we eat too much, still feel hungry and eat sweet things to combat the hunger pangs. And if we succumb to the promises made by the chocolate industry as well, their products just spoil the appetite and top up our fat reserves. The stomach problems that people experience show that stomach acid production has got completely out of control, while other factors exacerbating these problems include stress and smoking. This combination of symptoms may have only been prevalent among business managers some twenty years ago, but it has now become widespread in every class in society.

Reflex zones won't bring about any changes in behaviour, but at least they provide a means of soothing the stomach slightly.

1. Hand reflex zones
Stomach pain always seems to strike when you're out and about and the remedy is back home, sitting in a drawer, but fortunately all you need are your hands, which can be used discreetly to relieve many everyday complaints.

It's impossible to miss the stomach zone on the hand. If you press your thumb against your index finger, a small muscle rises on the back of the hand, to the rear of the thumb; release the fingers, massage this reflex zone area thoroughly and treat the maximum release points with basic unblocking. This reflex zone point is the same as an acupressure point used in China to achieve similar relief.

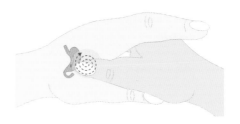

2. Foot reflex zones

For chronic and repetitive stomach problems, always see a doctor, but otherwise, reflex zone massage of the feet can help to improve the underlying situation. The area to treat is the solar plexus of the autonomic nervous system, which determines the wellness or otherwise of the upper abdomen. After a good, full massage of both feet, make exploratory circular strokes in the region around the solar plexus reflex zone. Basic unblocking of the most sensitive points will often uncover any tension relief that may have been delayed, but the beneficial effects will last a long time.

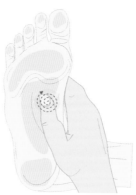

Complementary techniques

The stomach is actually a rather good-natured and forgiving organ that excuses many of our dietary mistakes, but if we overdo things with stress, nicotine and alcohol, as well as a bad diet, it can react with dyspepsia. The best way to treat this is by making changes to your diet and lifestyle. Herbal teas can also help to soothe this kind of complaint. Try a tea made from 20g peppermint, 25g camomile, 25g yarrow and 30g angelica root (leave to infuse in hot water for round 10 minutes; drink two cups daily for three weeks).

If heartburn is a persistent problem, it can be alleviated within minutes with just a small piece of raw potato, about the size of the tip of your thumb – but make sure you chew it well. In terms of essential oils, cumin and vetiver or cardamom are recommended in reflex zone massage, while the best gemstones to use are chalcedony, dolomite and citrine. Ultimately, the stomach is concerned with pleasure, and top chefs complain that we are gradually forgetting this.

Stress in the workplace

The invention of the typewriter placed great strain on people working on them seated at a desk. Unfortunately, the arrival of the computer did little to make things better, merely changing the situation rather than improving it; the physical demands on the hands and fingers as they pounded away at a mechanical keyboard have simply given way to the shoulder and neck problems associated with screen work.

A lack of motivation can also be a problem, such as when you're sitting at your desk with a task that should have been finished some time ago still in front of you, but instead you're fiddling with a biro or staring out into space. When motivation is lacking, it's hard to concentrate on the task at hand and piles of documents have a tendency to remain untouched. This is where the reflex zones come in. The hand zones can be used to help combat tension, while massage applied behind the ears and a finger workout accompanied by a breathing exercise should be sufficient to give you a new lease of life and spur you on to get down to work again.

1. Hand reflex zones

It's possible to carry out these massages discreetly in the office. After making soft circular strokes deep into the balls of your thumbs, work through your finger joints to loosen up the muscles of your shoulders.

Now it's time to turn your attention to your neck muscles.

Massage the cervical spine zones on the inner side of the thumb, using gentle circular strokes from top to bottom and applying basic unblocking to any sensitive points.

The 'grip' to improve motivation makes use of the brain zones, located in the fingertips. Simply place the fingertips together and gently massage them against one another, breathing in and out deeply three or four times.

2. Ear reflex zones

Many people pull at their earlobes when they are concentrating, and this is exactly where the brain zones are located – further proof that we intuitively make use of the reflex zones we need. These simple ear techniques will help you to use these zones to improve your motivation, concentration and memory: rub the earlobe well between thumb and index finger, making circular movements to massage the reflex zones – remembering of course that even when the massage is quite intense, it should always be pleasant. Finish by stroking as if you were trying to stretch the earlobe gently.

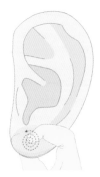

Complementary techniques

Two factors are key to ensuring wellbeing seated at a desk in the work environment: the atmosphere in the room or office and the seat or chair you are sitting on. A difficult atmosphere at work creates stress, while a poor sitting posture places strain on the entire musculoskeletal system. Office work should therefore be counterbalanced with some sports, such as Nordic walking or fitness training, both of which are particularly suitable. A relaxing holiday during which you can unwind fully is also an important part of restoring mental balance.

Essential oils (frankincense, marjoram, rosemary and cypress) can be used as a complement to reflex zone massage, while a diluted blend of these also makes a good massage oil for tension in the shoulders and neck. In terms of gemstones, red jasper and amethyst are particularly effective, as they bring energy to these regions. The reflex zones on the neck line (see 'Headaches', page 49) further complement the two techniques for the hands and ears.

Toothache

There's no need to be scared of the dentist – we might have some pain before a dental treatment and sometimes even afterwards, but, thanks to local anaesthetic, it is really only likely to be fear that we feel when seated in the dentist's surgery. Reflex zones have often been used with success to relieve discomfort before an appointment or after dental work has been carried out, but do consult your dentist without delay if you have any dental problems.

Techniques applied to the hands and ears can do more, however: they also promote lymph drainage and so can help the swelling associated with many dental treatments to subside more quickly.

The reflex zones of the ear and hand can be used for all problems affecting the oral cavity, from helping with cold sores on the lips to soothing a hoarse or sore throat. The essential technique in this case is almost always basic unblocking, which may take a little longer with problems of this kind. And, as ever, remember that it's important to always keep the treatment pleasant.

1. Hand reflex zones

The reflex zones responsible for the teeth are located in the regions above and below the metacarpophalangeal joints of the fingers, with the zones for the teeth of the upper jaw located on the back of the hand and those for the lower jaw on the palm.

For this treatment, make circular movements to explore the whole area and to search out any sensitive points; basic unblocking should be carried out wherever an unpleasant reflex zone point pops up. You may find that one or two of these points react particularly intensely; these maximum release points will often only subside after one or two repetitions about 15 minutes apart.

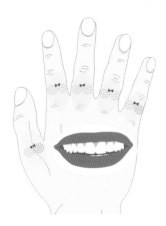

2. Ear reflex zones

This reflex zone system offers great potential for pain relief caused by dental problems and it is fascinating just how quick and long-lasting the effects on toothache can be.

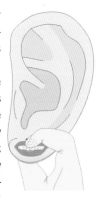

The zones for this technique are located in the area connecting the earlobe to the ear cavity. As you will almost certainly find that these zones are sensitive, apply the massage only very cautiously and sometimes it may not be possible to unblock them at the first attempt; some relief is generally experienced after the second or third basic unblocking (carried out at 15-minute intervals). Finish with gentle effleurage of the ears.

Complementary techniques

All dentists recommend the same regime: good dental care, avoiding food and liquid that is too hot or too cold on the teeth, cold compresses on the cheek for swelling, and taking painkillers as required. In many cases analgesics can be replaced with reflex zone treatment and in an emergency the mouth can be rinsed with a solution of oil of cloves (1–2 drops in a glass of water). Healing crystal therapy teaches us that sugilite, a very beautiful violet gemstone, can soothe toothache; it can be bought as tumbled stones at any good gemstone store. Ultimately, however, the best complementary therapy for dental problems is taking good care of your teeth and having them looked after and checked by a qualified professional.

Women's health

Women generally take more care of their health than men, live longer and have a greater tolerance to pain. However, many women have problems with their periods, and monthly bleeding is often accompanied by a sense of unease and abdominal tension, while menopausal problems include sweating, inner disquiet and listlessness.

Each woman develops her own strategy for coping with menstruation and fortunately many women have no problems at all, indeed quite the opposite: some experience an increase in their physical and mental well-being, and the same is true of the menopause. Some women even describe this period of hormonal readjustment as a blessing, but they are somewhat in the minority; for many women, the menopause is fraught with extreme mood swings and strong physical reactions. In such circumstances, the reflex zones can help to alleviate the basic situation and provide support on difficult days.

1. Hand reflex zones
If there were a reflex zone chart of 'hits', this hand treatment would be at the top – it is discreet and highly effective.

The reflex zones for the entire abdomen are located in the area around the base of the hand, at the wrist. When feeling unwell with

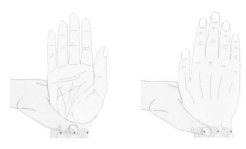

abdominal tension during periods and the menopause, use firm yet pleasant strokes from side to side across both sides of the wrists. Follow these with circular movements and if these reveal any sensitive points, they can be relieved with basic unblocking, which will, in turn, relieve tension in the body.

2. Back reflex zones

We're familiar with the location of these reflex zones, too – we hold our backs wherever we feel a pain, or tightness or stiffness. In terms of abdominal discomfort, it is also these zones that deal with the hormonal and reproductive organs.

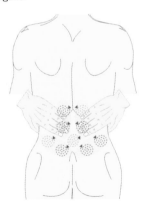

To soothe complaints affecting these areas, begin by making parallel, circular strokes across the sacrum with both hands. Make three or four circles at each point, as far as the pliability of the skin will allow, then move a circle higher. Slowly work up the back in this fashion; devote more attention to massaging any particularly sensitive zones and, to finish, lay your hands on the skin and take a few long breaths.

Complementary techniques

Women who experience problems during menstruation need peace and quiet and for their period generally to be a stress-free time. A herbal tea made with 20g St John's wort, 20g yarrow, 20g lemon balm, 20g tansy, 10g birch leaves and 10g rosemary relieves tension during a period and will also help during the menopause, when it stabilises the mood (drink two to three cups of the tea for around three weeks, then take a six-week break before taking the tea again for another three weeks). Homeopathic remedies provide an all-round complement to this treatment.

A nice warm bath or a soothing hot water bottle placed on the stomach is always helpful for menstrual complaints. A few drops of geranium, jasmine or lavender oil increase the effectiveness of the bath or, alternatively, rub some of the diluted oil into the stomach and place a small, damp flannel on the skin underneath a hot water bottle. These oils are also used in reflex zone massage. Suitable crystals for gemstone massage for period pains include tumbled stones of serpentine, malachite or amber, while tiger eye and garnet can also be used during the menopause.

Guide to the reflex zones charts

The charts on the following pages indicate where to find the right reflex zone for the part of the body you wish to treat – for example, your right shoulder, may be troubling you, or perhaps you want some relief for a nagging upper left wisdom tooth, which is due to be extracted tomorrow. To use the charts, you just need to follow the three hand zone rules:

1. **Left–right rule:** the reflex zones for all the organs on the right side of the body are to be found on the right hand and those on the left side of the body on the left hand. To find the dividing line down the centre of the body, hold your thumbs together, adjacent to one another. So the zone for that problematic right shoulder is at the far edge of the right hand, and the zone for that troublesome wisdom tooth is between the left middle and ring finger.

2. **Front–back rule:** the reflex zones for all the organs at the front of the body, such as the nose or stomach, are on the back of the hand and all the organs at the back of the body, such as the neck or the backside, are represented on the other (palm) side of the hand. The inner organs and the joints can be accessed on both sides of the hands. So that painful shoulder joint and the doomed wisdom tooth are represented in zones both on the back of the hand and the palm.

3. **Level rule:** the body is represented in the hand reflex zones like a three-dimensional picture; the reference points are the spinal segments.

Skull	Fingertips	Brain
Cervical spine	Proximal phalanges of the fingers	Sensory organs, oral cavity, teeth, throat, neck, tonsils
Thoracic spine	Metacarpals	Heart, lung, liver, gall bladder, pancreas, spleen
Lumbar spine	Carpals	Bowel, kidneys, bladder, reproductive organs
Sacrum, coccyx	Wrist joint	Pelvic floor, hip

When looking for the reflex zones relating to a specific problem, picture your body in terms of the hand image to find the relevant area: the zone for the right shoulder is located on the metacarpophalangeal joint of the little finger and the zone for the tooth is between that joint and the next finger joint.

Once you have found the target area, you can narrow down the exact reflex zone points by noting their sensitivity or unpleasant sensations and treat them accordingly.

INNER hand reflex zones

Brain

Ears

Oral cavity

Thyroid/
throat

Stomach

Liver

Pancreas

Small
intestine

Kidney

Reproductive
organs

Hand

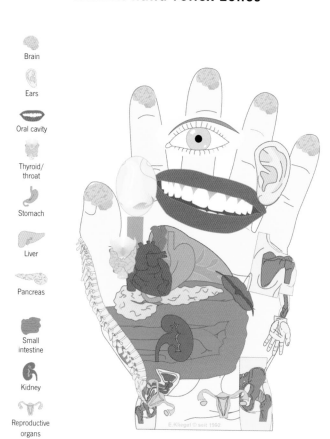

E.Kliegel © seit 1992

INNER hand reflex zones

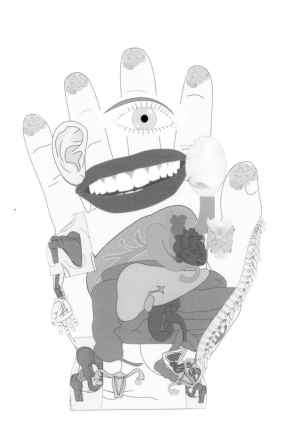

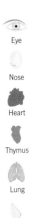
Eye

Nose

Heart

Thymus

Lung

Mammary gland

Spleen

Large intestine

Bladder

Shoulder

Hip

Elbow

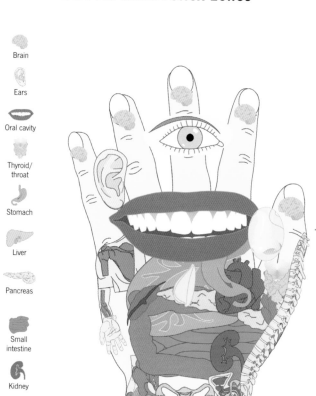

Brain

Ears

Oral cavity

Thyroid/
throat

Stomach

Liver

Pancreas

Small
intestine

Kidney

Reproductive
organs

Hand

OUTER hand reflex zones

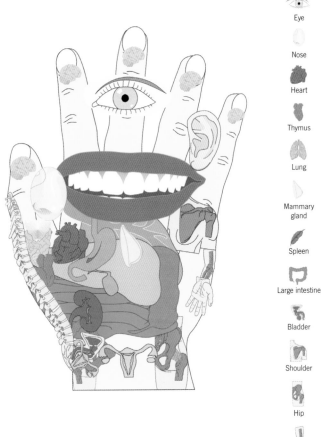

Eye

Nose

Heart

Thymus

Lung

Mammary gland

Spleen

Large intestine

Bladder

Shoulder

Hip

Elbow

About the author

Ewald Kliegel (b. 1957)

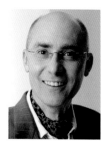

Ewald Kliegel's professional engagement with people began in 1976, when he took up two internships – one in a urology clinic and the other in a school for children with learning disabilities. Since then, his life has been devoted to the twin topics of healing and teaching, while his medical training as a masseur and naturopath have paved the way to a holistic perspective on body and soul. He has been teaching at alternative therapy schools and in his own seminars in Germany and abroad since 1989.

In his 'Reflexology: Maps of Health' (Landkarten der Gesundheit), published in 1992, Ewald Kliegel established a coherent formal vocabulary for depicting more than thirty reflex zone systems, while in 1996, he introduced crystal wands as tools developed for reflex zone treatment and acupressure. Around 1999, he began research for his book 'Reflex Zones and the Language of the Organs' (Reflexzonen und Organsprache), published in 2008, in which a series of diverting stories portray the organs not as sites of illness but rather as archetypal pictures of the soul that affect our innermost being. Taking this idea even further, he placed the organs at the spiritual and emotional centre of our being, where they reveal their true selves and the concept underlying their creation. Ann Heng has illustrated Ewald Kliegel's book 'Let Your Body Speak' (Findhorn Press) with her superb images.

In the seminars in his 'reflex-balance' programme, Ewald Kliegel teaches courses in reflex zone and gemstone treatment for use in therapy and professional wellness sessions. He also gives lectures and holds seminars and events to awaken our organs to their psycho-spiritual capabilities, in which a healing zone for a deep connection with the body's organs can be created through self-awareness, mindfulness and meditational devotion. These events and seminars are suitable for professional work with patients, as well as for improving one's own physical self-awareness or as a precautionary psycho-spiritual measure for promoting good health.

Contact:

Ewald Kliegel
Rotenbergstr. 154
70190 Stuttgart
Germany
info@reflex-balance.eu

Consult our catalogue online (with secure order facility) on
www.findhornpress.com
Earthdancer Books is an Imprint of Findhorn Press.
www.earthdancer.co.uk

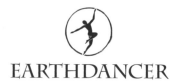

A FINDHORN PRESS IMPRINT